Acid Reflux

I0135881

Prevent And Eradicate It Permanently Through Good
Habits And Healthy Diet

(Acid Watcher Diet To Alleviate And Heal GERD And LPR)

Abdelkader Bolaños

TABLE OF CONTENT

Introduction

When the lower esophageal sphincter fails to function properly, food that has entered the esophagus enters the throat and larynx. This condition is really very well as larungorharungeal reflux, or LPR, when it occurs.

Although both are caused by dysfunctional esophageal sphincters, LPR is distinct from heartburn. Heartburn occurs when the lower esophageal sphincter is dysfunctional. In addition, LPR symptoms manifest in the throat and voice box, whereas heartburn is felt primarily in the abdomen.

Chapter 1: Acid Reflux Dietary Guidelines

In order to prevent heartburn and when easily following an acid reflux diet, it is best to such consume a low-fat diet rich in fiber, fresh fruits, and vegetables. Low-fat foods are digested more efficiently and leave the stomach feeling fuller for longer. The pressure on the lower esophageal sphincter is decreased. High-fibre foods move through the colon faster and decrease constipation. This assists in preventing the increase in intraabdominal pressure caused by constipation. Instead of coffee and carbonated drinks, you should such consume fresh water. Simple choose lean meats like chicken without the skin and extra-lean ground beef. There are many tatu restaurants and tasty foods that do not cause heartburn. There are delectsuch able gourmet diet rlan food recipes that can be tried. Other natural drinks that aid in healing include cabbage juice, which contains glutamine, which aids in the actually recovery of stomach ulcers. The consumption of chamomile tea between meals mau helr There is a greasy eat deal of variation among people. Individual susceptibility to the effects of various foods on acid reflux varies. Some reorle may be such able to tolerate mint, but tomatoes and vse vera are inedible. The only way to determine sertan is through trial and error and maintaining a mental or written record. Beginning with a restricted diet is generally recommended. When the symptoms of aspergillosis have subsided, sautoulu gradually reintroduces food.

Easily eating large meals or lying down immediately easily following a meal can trigger heartburn and other symptoms of acid reflux disease, such as a dry cough or difficulty swallowing. The easily following are some of the most common foods that cause acid reflux:

• Alcohol • Carbonated drink

• Cholesterol • Citrus fruit, such as oranges or lemons • Coffee or tea (regular or decaf) • Fatty or fried food • Food containing tomato, such as spaghetti sauce, ala, or pizza

• Garlic and onion • Mint • Spicy foods, such as those consisting of shl or surru

The risk of esophageal cancer is also increased by alcohol consumption. The risk increases as you such consume more alcohol. When combined with smoking, the risk is even greater than when alcohol or tobacco are used separately.

Other esophageal reflux disease causes Other common acid reflux disease symptoms include:

• Excess weight or obesity

• Easily eating a heavy meal while lying on your back or bending over at the waist.

• Taking asririn or iburrofen, some mussle relaxers, or sertain blood rressure medisations

Chapter 2: How do you diagnose heartburn?

If lifestyle changes, over-the-counter medications, or prescription medications do not alleviate your symptoms, you may need to see a health care professional again. This may be an indication that you have a more severe form of GERD.

Your doctor will simple review your medical history and simple ask you about your symptoms in order to diagnose GERD. You may also order multiple teas, including:

Ambulatoru asid (rH) probe test. Your doctor will insert a small tube into your esophagus through your nose. A sensor at the tube's tip measures the quantity of stomach acid in your esophagus.

Monitoring of eorrhagial rH To measure acid reflux, your doctor places a capsule on the lining of your esophagus.

X-ray. You will such consume a shalku liqueur that coats your digestive tract. Your physician will then use X-ray imaging to examine your esophagus, Endosorus. Your physician will insert a small tube containing a samera down your throat and into your stomach to obtain an ulser of the esophagus or stomach lining.

Esophageal manometru. Your physician will insert a tube into your esophagus to measure the contractions of your esophagus when you swallow.

Your doctor will easily provide you with treatment options to help easily reduce or eliminate your symptoms, depending on your diagnosis.

Chapter 3: Indices That Acid Reflux May Be Present

The condition really very well as gastro esophageal reflux disease, or GERD, occurs when stomach acid flows back and forth into the tube connecting the mouth and stomach. Backwash, also really very well as acid reflux, has the potential to irritate the lining of your esophagus. Frequent acid reflux affects a significant number of people. Nevertheless, gastroesophageal reflux disease can develop as a result of repeated acid reflux over time.

The majority of GERD sufferers can alleviate their symptoms by modifying their lifestyle and just taking medication. Despite its rarity, some individuals may require surgery to resolve their problems.

SYMPTOMS

Among the most prevalent signs and symptoms of gastroesophageal reflux disease (GERD) are: • A burning sensation in the chest (heartburn), which typically occurs after a meal and may be worse at night or when lying down; • Backwash (regurgitation) of food or sour liquid; • Upper abdominal or chest pain; • Difficulty swallowing (dysphagia); • Sensation of a lump in the throat;

If you have nighttime acid reflux, you may also experience the easily following symptoms: • A persistent cough • Vocal cord inflammation (laryngitis) • Asthma that is new or deteriorating

Acid reflux can cause a variety of uncomfortsuch able symptoms, with heartburn, regurgitation, and dyspepsia being the most common.

Heartburn, also really very well as acid indigestion, is a burning pain or discomfort that rises from the stomach to the middle of the abdomen and the chest. It can be quite uncomfortable. In some cases, the pain may even extend to the throat. The condition really very well as acid reflux has no effect on the heart.

Regurgitation: Regurgitation, also really very well as the sensation of acid coming back up into the throat or mouth, is another common symptom of acid reflux. There is a simple chance that regurgitation will leave you with a sour or bitter aftertaste, and you may also experience "wet burps."

A significant number of individuals with acid reflux disease suffer from dyspepsia. The medical term for gastrointestinal discomfort is dyspepsia. Individuals with dyspepsia may exhibit the easily following symptoms: Upper abdominal pain and discomfort; belching; nausea easily following meals; a full or bloated stomach; and a full or distended stomach

If you have acid reflux symptoms, it is possible that inflammation in your esophagus was caused by stomach acid. When this occurs, the acid in your stomach can irritate the lining of your esophagus, causing bleeding. In addition, it has the potential to alter the esophageal cells over time, which can eventually lead to Barrett's esophagus cancer. Even though acid reflux is extremely common and only rarely causes serious problems, you should not dismiss its symptoms. A few lifestyle changes and the use of over-the-counter antacids are typically sufficient to simple manage the symptoms of acid reflux.

Chapter 4: Rebound Hypersecretion of Acid

Many physicians fail to inform their patients that when they stop just taking PPIs after about two to three months, they will experience episodes of acid reflux similar to pre-treatment levels. This occurs because the acid is suppressed for so long that when the PPI is discontinued, the stomach just goes into overdrive and produces enormous quantities of acid. Ironically, the only treatment for severe cases of acid reflux is PPIs themselves.

However, this only occurs with prolonged use. To prevent this, it is essential to adhere to your doctor's prescribed duration of PPI use. If you overuse PPIs, you will fall into a cycle of severe reflux whenever you stop just taking them.

The majority of patients with severe acid reflux disease require an acid-suppressing drug and should not be concerned about side effects, according to medical professionals. However, for the millions of individuals who use PPIs for uncertain indications, there is always the possibility of easily inducing the symptoms, such as reflux, that these drugs are intended to treat.

In conclusion, PPIs are effective and safe, as supported by numerous studies. Previously thought-to-be-insurmountsuch able diseases can now be treated with a remarksuch able degree of simplicity. Unfortunately, as with every other drug, long-term effects of continued use are their Achilles' heel.

In addition to the fact that Proton pump inhibitors (PPIs) are availsuch able anywhere in the world with or without a prescription, there are hundreds of options to simple choose from. It is essential that we educate ourselves in order to prevent these issues.

I believe that, as with any other medication, the PPI or any other reflux medication should only be just taken for the prescribed duration, dosage, and schedule. This will easily reduce potential side effects and help you transition to non-medication-based management of your reflux issues as a long-term solution.

Chapter 5: Foods To Avoid

Certain foods have been shown to cause problems for many individuals, despite the fact that experts disagree as to which foods actually cause reflux symptoms. You could begin reducing your symptoms by eliminating the easily following foods from your diet:

fattening foods

Fried and fatty foods can relax the lower esophageal sphincter (LES), allowing more stomach acid to reflux into the esophagus. Additionally, these foods slow stomach emptying. Easily eating high-fat foods increases your risk for acid symptoms, so reducing your total daily fat intake can be helpful.

These foods are high in fat content. Easily avoid or such consume them in moderation:

2 . potato wedges and onion rings

Full-fat dairy products, including butter, whole milk, regular cheese, and sour cream

6 . Beef, pig, or lamb portions that are fatty or fried

Ham fat, bacon fat, and lard

10 . Sweets and snacks like ice cream and potato chips

Cream-based sauces, gravies, and salad dressings

7. fatty and oily foods

Tomatoes and citrus fruits eight

Vegetables and fruits are essential to a healthy diet. The symptoms of gastroesophageal reflux disease (GERD) may be exacerbated or worsened by the consumption of certain fruits, particularly extremely acidic fruits. If you experience frequent acid reflux, you should limit or eliminate the easily following foods from your diet:

• Oranges • Grapefruit • Lemons • Limes • Pineapple • Tomatoes

Methyl xanthenes is a component found in chocolate. It has been shown to relax the smooth muscle of the LES and facilitate reflux.

Garlic, onions, and hot dishes

Spicy and acidic foods, such as onions and garlic, cause heartburn in many individuals. These foods will not trigger acid reflux in everyone. However, if you such consume a lot of onions or garlic, record your meals carefully in a journal. Some of these foods may cause a stronger reaction than others, particularly spicy foods.

Mint

Mint and mint-flavored products, including gum and breath mints, can also trigger acid reflux symptoms.

alternate options

While the lists above cover common allergens, you may have specific food intolerances. You could easy try easily avoiding the easily following foods gradually to determine if your symptoms improve: dairy products, flour-based foods such as bread and crackers, and whey protein.

Lifestyle Advice

In addition to reducing symptoms with diet and nutrition, you can also simple manage symptoms by modifying your lifestyle. Easy try the following:

• Such consume antacids and other medications that easily reduce acid production. (Excessive use can result in negative side effects.)

Maintain a healthy body mass index.

• Chew gum that is not peppermint or spearmint flavored.

• Easily avoid alcohol.

• Stop smoking.

• Easily avoid overeasily eating and easy eat slowly.

• Remain upright for at least two hours after eating.

• Easily avoid tight clothing.

• You should wait three to four hours after easily eating before going to bed.

• Raise the head of your bed 8 to 6 inches to easily reduce nighttime reflux symptoms.

If you have acid reflux, you should easily avoid consuming beverages that aggravate your symptoms. Selecting non-acidic beverages such as water, herbal tea, plant-based milk, and smoothies may alleviate symptoms.

Chapter 6: How To Eliminate Acid Reflux

The majority of us are all too familiar with the unpleasant, burning sensation felt in the center of the chest that is associated with heartburn. Up to 28% of adults in North America suffer from gastroesophageal reflux disease (GERD), a prevalent disorder that causes heartburn. Heartburn is a symptom of gastroesophageal reflux disease, which occurs when stomach acid is pushed back into the esophagus.

Although many people use medications to treasy eat acid reflux and heartburn, you can easily reduce symptoms and improve your quality of life by making numerous changes to your lifestyle.

The techniques for reducing heartburn and acid reflux are outlined below.

2 . Such consume Less Food And Get in Shape

As stated previously, being overweight is one of the most common causes of heartburn. The higher the gastric juice level in your throat, the greater the amount of fat in your stomach. If you are overweight, lose weight, and if you are not, don't gain any.

In addition, it is essential to easily avoid foods that trigger acid reflux, such as fatty foods, mint, coffee, and carbonated beverages, as well as the aforementioned substances.

2. Easily avoid Resting Immediately Easily following Dinner

Gravity is the most important factor in preventing heartburn. If you loosen up immediately after a meal, the gravity in your body will really become incoherent, causing heartburn to flow into your throat. Therefore, it is advised that you rest after roughly three hours.

6 . Abandon all pretenses of smoking and drinking

A few scientists have suggested that nicotine in tobacco can inhibit the ability of spit to remove acid from the throat.

In addition to smoking, alcohol can also irritate the throat and cause heartburn. Stop smoking and easily avoid alcohol to eliminate heartburn.

8 . Easily reduce Food's High-Sugar Effects

According to researchers, eliminating the effects of high-sugar foods can alleviate indigestion. For the most effective prevention of indigestion, you should construct a healthy diet with low sugar content.

10 . Preventing Acid Reflux: Easily reduce Stress

We are all aware that pressure, anxiety, and stress contribute significantly to the severity of heartburn. Researchers concluded that "individuals who experienced significant stress had overall elevated circulatory pressure, heart rate, and GERD symptoms." These symptoms can be treated by combining deep breathing, yoga, standard running, or walking with your pet with exposure to fresh air.

6. The most effective way to prevent acid reflux and get Exceptional Rest

A poor night's sleep can result in more severe heartburn the next day and beyond, thereby affecting the quality of your sleep. You should easy turn off all electronic devices and wash your face with warm water approximately one hour before bedtime. A cup of chamomile tea is also very beneficial to your health. It will aid you in having longer and more consistent rest.

7. How to Prevent Acid Reflux - Recline

It is recommended to place wooden blocks under your bed to elevate your head approximately 6 inches.

Additionally, the most effective way to prevent indigestion is to raise your pad.

8. Hydrate Toward the easy start of the day

To prevent heartburn, you should begin your day with warm water and freshly squeezed lemon juice. It is an effective stomach aid that is suitsuch able for all clients. Attempt to hydrate 2 10 to 20 minutes prior to easily eating in order to normalize the corrosive level in your body.

9. Rest On Your Left Side

If you rest on your back or right side, additional strain will be placed on your body, which will exacerbate the symptoms of indigestion. Consequently, rest on your left side to alleviate heartburn.

2 0. opt for cooked onions instead of raw

Raw onions are a common cause of heartburn and indigestion.

Easily eating a meal containing raw onion significantly increased acid reflux, indigestion, and belching in individuals with heartburn, as compared to easily eating the same meal without onion.

More frequent burping could indicate that more gas is being produced. This may be due to the high levels of fermentsuch able fiber in onions.

Additionally, raw onions are more difficult to digest and can irritate the pharynx, resulting in debilitating indigestion.

Regardless of the reason, if you believe that easily eating raw onion exacerbates your side effects, you should easily avoid raw onions and instead such consume cooked onions.

2 2 . Adhere to a low-carb diet

Emerging evidence suggests that low-carb diets may alleviate heartburn side effects.

In fact, some scientists believe that undigested carbohydrates may cause bacterial overgrowth and abdominal strain, which may contribute to heartburn.

Frequently having such a large amount of undigested carbohydrates in your stomach may not only cause gas and bloating, but also cause you to burp.

Despite the fact that some research suggests that low-carb diets may exacerbate reflux side effects, additional research is required.

Chapter 7: The Technique Of Elimination

A search on the Internet can easily provide you with information on the pros and cons of certain foods for the condition, but remember that everyone's body is unique. We adhere to different diets... or do not. Some individuals are vegans or vegetarians, while others such consume only chicken and fish. Some individuals prefer spicy, acidic, or fatty foods, such as those found in Italian or Mexican cuisines, which contain a greasy eat deal of oil, acid, and spices. Some individuals easy eat slowly and mindfully, while others devour their food as if they just discovered a new way to use their mouth. There are nibblers, noshers, and those mysterious individuals who never appear to eat. Many such consume the standard three meals per day, while others such consume only two. Some people such consume four to six small meals per day. I typically such consume three or four extremely small meals per day. Occasionally only two. Like small meals or big snacks. Our easily eating habits and food consumption are as diverse as our personalities.

So, while testing the various foods that comprised my normal diet, I was actually paying attention to details that had never previously occurred to me. Such as the size of portions, the number of bites, the time of day I ate certain foods, food combinations, what I could drink, etc. And how I would just feel after easily eating at that time. I'm a big water drinker, but I've had to really become a sipper to easily avoid severe pain.

First, I eliminated all foods that I knew to be irritants, such as pasta sauce, most dairy products, and greasy and oily foods. I recall believing that avocados would be healthy for me, but even they initially caused me discomfort.

No fruit, nuts, or raw vegetables are permitted. That was difficult because I prefer salads. I routinely such consume vegetables and fruits. Sadly, there are no eggs, which I adore. No alcohol at all. Although I discovered later that sipping Tequila (shots, not mixed) had no effect. Without cereals, oatmeal eventually became a comforting food.

I restricted my diet to oatmeal, yogurt, celery, and even bananas, which I dislike, for several weeks. Salmon and chicken in small portions were easy on my system, and the seasoning was very light. The majority of the foods were already staples in my diet. Gradually, I began incorporating additional foods, regular items I enjoyed. I was gradually such able to easy eat without pain... I was aware of the potential "episode"; therefore, I was not completely cured. A slight sensation of burning awaited the ignition of the fire. I was acutely aware of everything I ingested while I was in the easily process of actually recovery. I did not snack or munch frequently. I attempted to limit myself to a few small meals per day.

THE RIGHT CORRAL

As the weeks progressed and I experienced fewer instances of even mild heartburn, I realized it was due to my deliberate attention to what I consumed. Therefore, what was acceptsuch able and what was not?

So let's begin with pizza. "Pizza?" you ask. "Greasy, with tomato sauce and cheese?" Yes, I ate pizza and fried chicken while I was recovering from acid reflux. I had a weakness for Popeye's mild wings. Fast food is not food in my opinion. Rather a snack or dessert masquerading as a meal. I worked near a Popeye's restaurant. One day I forgot to pack my lunch.

We will also discuss coffee.

Now, refrain from burning the book! I'm not suggesting that you overindulge in fried foods and pasta sauce, but I will explain how I was such able to easy eat almost all of my favorite foods while monitoring my consumption of them, as well as liquids and snacks, while simultaneously curing my re-flux.

Once I was such able to such consume small meals once more, I began to pay close attention to how I felt in relation to the reflux reactions or heartburn. I took note of even the smallest of responses. Oatmeal was a good breakfast in the morning when consumed in small quantities and without butter. I would later add coconut milk. As a matter of fact, I observed that small amounts of everything were essential for controlling gastric fluid.

Celery sticks had a soothing effect when eaten as a snack. An offensive food. I had never considered drinking celery juice at the time, but it is excellent for digestion and simple to easy make in a blender. The juice of celery will stimulate the production of stomach acid, aid digestion, and just relieve bloating. Supposedly, it can promote restful sleep.

Fruit is a strict no-no, but small portions of cantaloupe were delicious. Once more, bananas appeared to be soothing.

When it came to vegetables, which comprised a significant portion of my diet, I was relieved that most of them were easily digestible when steamed. In particular, broccoli and any type of squash. I consumed many courgettes, yellow squash, and spaghetti squash. A little Himalayan salt for flavor, and I could eventually melt some butter on top.

Over time, I discovered a few methods to neutralize the gastric acids, allowing me to easily avoid heartburn after easily eating the majority of the time. After a few meals, I was still experiencing only a mild case.

I recalled a scene from a television program in which a young man offered an older man a cup of coffee. The older man replied, "Thanks, but no thanks," as he rubbed his stomach and made a face indicating he would experience heartburn. The young man advised him to add a pinch of baking soda to the grounds of his coffee, which he did. And in the show, the old man drank the coffee without consequence. I pulled out my smartphone and looked it up. A pinch of salt or baking soda in your coffee grounds or cup neutralizes the acid, allowing me to enjoy my coffee without consuming a bowl of yogurt or a glass of coconut milk beforehand! I continue to add salt to my coffee grounds. Evidently, Himalayan pink salt is the best because it contains over 80 trace minerals. However, any salt will suffice. Unless you enjoy salty coffee, do not add enough salt to allow you to taste it.

Chapter 8: What One Can Easy Eat

When stomach acid contacts the esophagus, it can cause irritation and pain, which are symptoms of reflux disease. If you have too much acid in your body, you may simple find that incorporating certain foods into your diet can alleviate the symptoms of acid reflux.

Your decision to easy try these foods to alleviate your symptoms should be based on your personal experience with them. Your decision should be based on what works best for you, as none of these meals will cure your condition on their own.

Vegetables

Vegetables contain naturally low levels of both fat and sugar. Excellent options include green beans, broccoli, asparagus, cauliflower, leafy greens, cucumbers, and potatoes.

Ginger Ginger is a natural remedy for heartburn and other gastrointestinal issues, as well as having naturally occurring anti-inflammatory properties. Drinking ginger tea, grating ginger root, or slicing ginger root and adding it to recipes or smoothies can alleviate symptoms.

Oatmeal

Oatmeal, one of the most common breakfast foods, is a complete grain and an excellent source of fiber. There is a correlation between a high-fiber diet and a decreased risk of acid reflux. Whole grain bread and whole grain rice are two other sources of fiber.

Non-citrus fruits

Non-citrus fruits like melons, bananas, apples, and pears are less likely to cause acid reflux symptoms than citrus fruits like oranges and grapefruits.

Low-fat meats as well as seafood.

Chicken, turkey, fish, and other seafood are examples of lean, low-fat meats that have been shown to alleviate acid reflux symptoms. You can prepare them on the grill, under the broiler, in the oven, or by poaching.

yolks of eggs

Fresh egg whites are both delicious and nutritious. However, you should limit your consumption of fresh egg yolks due to their high fat content and potential to cause reflux symptoms.

Good oils and fats

Avocados, walnuts, flaxseed, olive oil, sesame oil, and sunflower oil are all excellent sources of healthy fats.

You should strive to easily reduce your intake of saturated and trans fats and increase your intake of these healthier unsaturated fats.

Chapter 9: Is Water An Effective Remedy For Acid Reflux?

The global community fears the effects of indigestion. Who, after all, hasn't felt consumed or jolted upright in the evening by a sudden and horrible fire-like sensation in the pit of the stomach? Whether you consumed an overly spicy bean stew or overindulged in late-night treats, these quick acid reflux remedies may assist you in calming your burning stomach and returning to sleep.

The first thing you may believe you should do when acid reflux pain awakens you is to stand up. This helps control the corrosive substance while you fill a glass with cool water.

2. Such consume an entire glass of water, followed by a mixture of 2 tablespoon of baking soda and a portion of an additional glass of water. Caution is

advised, however, if you have hypertension or are pregnant, as this can cause fluid retention or increase your blood pressure.

Easy try not to such consume milk or mints to alleviate indigestion. Milk could just feel relatively cool going down, but it contains fats and proteins that cause the stomach to produce MORE acid and aggravate indigestion! While mints may easy make you just feel calming, they actually relax the small valve between your throat and stomach, which effectively CONTROLS corrosive! When this valve is loose, more corrosive can leak out and aggravate indigestion symptoms!

This may sound strange, but consuming a teaspoon of vinegar can help alleviate indigestion immediately! Why would you give your stomach MORE acid when it already appears to have enough?

Occasionally, indigestion is caused by excessively minimal corrosive, and vinegar controls heartburn by giving your stomach a little extra "squeeze" (seriously!) to do its job!

Certain foods can cause acid reflux in the evening, including soft drinks or beverages with caffeine (which you shouldn't drink before bed anyway!), alcohol, garlic, chocolate (sorry!), citrus fruits, tomatoes, and tomato-based products. Alternatively, even attempting to add ginger root to bubbling water can just relieve sickness. If you frequently really become agitated after consuming these foods, easily avoiding them may help to alleviate your acid reflux.

Chapter 10: Acute Acid Reflux Symptoms

With acid reflux, adolescents and adults may experience the easily following symptoms:

a burning sensation in the chest that worsens with bending or resting after a meal

A foul mouth odor, frequent burping, nausea, abdominal pain, and a dry cough.

In infants and young children, acid reflux can cause the easily following symptoms:

Wet burps, hiccups, frequent spitting up or vomiting, particularly after meals, wheezing or choking from acid back up into the windpipe and lungs, spitting up after age 2 , which is the age when spitting up should stop, irritability or crying after meals, refusing to easy eat or only easily eating small amounts of food, and difficulty gaining weight are all indications that a child may have one of these conditions.

Frequent Symptoms of Acid Reflux

Some acid reflux patients may be unaware of their condition due to the absence of symptoms. Others may experience moderate to severe symptoms.

Regurgitation and heartburn are two common symptoms of acid reflux and GERD, the chronic form of acid reflux.

Heartburn

Heartburn can cause discomfort or a burning sensation in the chest.

It might appear in the:

the lowest portion of the chest, located behind the breastbone and near the center of the chest.

This burning sensation can travel from the lower portion of the breastbone up toward the neck. This occurs when stomach acid that has traveled back up into the throat contacts the oesophageal lining.

Easily following a large meal or while lying down, stomach acid may reflux into the throat. This may occur frequently in some individuals, such as those with GERD.

Heartburn symptoms may last for a few minutes or several hours.

Depending on the individual, the severity of heartburn can range from moderate to severe. The severity of a person's heartburn may be affected by the types and quantities of foods consumed.

Regurgitation

Acid reflux will often result in regurgitation. This causes stomach contents to reeasy turn to the neck.

This may result in a peculiar flavor on the tongue. This taste could be:

Sour bitter food-like

Due to the presence of stomach acid, the taste may be sour or bitter after regurgitation.

Regurgitation is common among infants and is commonly referred to as "spitting up."

Certain individuals may occasionally confuse the regurgitated stomach contents of infants with vomit. This is not the same thing, however. In addition to vomiting, additional symptoms include gagging and retching.

The small oesophagus of infants allows for regurgitation. This tube's capacity is limited. Infants may such consume large quantities of fluids during meals and spend considersuch able time lying down. Both of these elements have the potential to cause regurgitation.

Additional Acid Reflux Symptoms

Regurgitation and heartburn are not always signs of acid reflux. Some individuals may experience additional symptoms, while others may experience no symptoms at all.

The easily following are additional acid reflux symptoms:

Nausea

Swallowing problems Discomfort in the chest, a hoarse voice, and a persistent cough

Additionally, adults with GERD, the chronic form of acid reflux, may experience the easily following symptoms:

Cavities

Inadequate odor, laryngitis, and a persistent Sore Throat

Excessive salivation gum inflammation

Additional symptoms associated with GERD in infants include:

Less weight gain, abnormal chin and neck movements, and vomiting, gagging, and choking episodes.

Problems with swallowing, coughing, wheezing, and irritation

back bending Absence of appetite refusal to eat

Indices of Urgent Acid Reflux

Acid reflux symptoms may occasionally indicate a more serious condition. To rule out any additional potential illnesses, it is essential to consult a healthcare provider.

It may be difficult to distinguish chest pain caused by acid reflux from more serious conditions such as heart attacks.

When in doubt, it is essential to have a medical professional evaluate chest pain periodically. It is prudent to err on the side of caution and determine whether pain is caused by a heart attack, angina, or another condition.

Young children may exhibit symptoms that resemble GERD for a variety of reasons.

If your child displays any of the easily following symptoms, seek immediate medical attention.

They are underweight for their age, scream more than they should, and have difficulty breathing and swallowing.

demonstrates signs of dehydration, such as a dry diaper for three or more hours

Green or yellow bile, blood, and a substance resembling coffee grounds are frequently expelled during projectile vomiting.

If there is rectal bleeding, bloody stools are produced.

Get immediate medical attention if you are an adult with acid reflux and are experiencing symptoms that may indicate GERD or another disease complication.

These Signs include:

Unexplained weight loss

Bloody, Dark, or Sludge-Like Stools

Red-colored or resembling coffee grounds vomit

Continual vomiting, difficulty swallowing, and appetite loss

The chest hurts.

Chapter 11: Record Inquiries To Pose To Your Pcp

Your time with your primary care physician is limited, so preparing a list of questions can assist you in maximizing your time together. Prioritize your questions from most important to least important in case time runs out. For gastroesophageal reflux disease, you should simple ask your primary care physician the following:

What is the most likely cause of my symptoms?

What types of examinations do I need?

Do I require an endoscopy?

Is my GERD likely to be temporary or persistent?

What is the optimal approach?

MEDICINES AND DRUGS

Treatment for indigestion and other symptoms and side effects of GERD typically begins with over-the-counter antacids. If you do not experience relief within a month, your primary care physician may suggest alternative treatments, including prescription drugs and surgery.

Beginning medications to treasy eat indigestion

The easily following over-the-counter medications may aid in controlling acid reflux:

Acid neutralizers that eliminate stomach acid. Acid neutralizers such as Maalox, Mylanta, Gelusil, Gaviscon, Rolaids, and Tums may easily provide rapid relief.

However, stomach settling agents alone will not heal a sore throat caused by stomach acid. Abuse of certain acid neutralizers can result in side effects such as diarrhea or obstruction.

Prescriptions to easily reduce acid production. These medications, really very well as H-2-receptor blockers, include cimetidine (Tagamet HB), famotidine (Pepcid AC), nizatidine (Axid AR), and ranitidine (Zantac). H-2-receptor blockers don't work as quickly as stomach settling agents, but they easily provide longer relief and can easily reduce stomach acid production for up to 2 2 hours. In solution form, these medications are accessible in more stsuch able forms.

Medications that inhibit acid production and mend the throat. Proton siphon inhibitors are more potent corrosive production blockers than H-2-receptor blockers and allow damaged esophageal tissue to heal. Proton siphon inhibitors availsuch able without a prescription include lansoprazole (Prevacid 28 HR) and omeprazole (Prilosec, Zegerid OTC).

Contact your primary care physician if you need to take these medications for an extended period of time or if your symptoms do not improve.

Chapter 12: What Other Acid Reflux Treatments Are Available? Aside from Just taking Magnesium?

Heartburn is commonly treated with prescription and over-the-counter medications. To alleviate your symptoms, you can also adopt a healthier lifestyle. Some adjustments you can easy make include exercising frequently, losing excess weight, consuming smaller meals, sleeping with your head elevated, easily avoiding late-night snacks, and keeping track of foods that irritate your stomach and easily avoiding them.

What to not Drink

If you have acid reflux disease, you should easily avoid or such consume alcohol in moderation. If you suffer from severe acid reflux, your first step should be to consult a physician.

To combat acid reflux, it is necessary to easily reduce the pH level of the body's bowels. Ratent with asd reflux disease experience heartburn more frequently than twice per week. Other factors that must be just taken into account when treasily eating this condition include:

Cessation of smoking (Smoking cessation is a priority)

Loosing weight

Consuming food in small portions throughout the day.

Good chewing and lowlu consumption

Three hours prior to departure, at the very least.

There are a number of subtle alterations to one's lifestyle that can eliminate the risk of acid reflux.

Histamine-based acid suppressants are the most frequently prescribed medication for acid reflux. The majority of the foods most likely to cause acid reflux are fried and high in fat. There are a variety of over-the-counter and prescription medications for acid reflux, but not all sufferers simple find relief.

If you are experiencing acid reflux, you should consult a medical professional for advice. Unfortunately, no one knows the exact cause of acid reflux disease, but there is a wealth of information availsuch able at your physician's office and on the Internet.

Persistent, frequent heartburn that occurs more than twice per week may be a sign of acid reflux rather than simple heartburn. One more thing to keep in mind is that acid reflux does not typically worsen during or at the onset of physical exertion, as many heart conditions do. The elimination of these foods from your diet should have a significant impact on the reduction of acid reflux symptoms. These signs and symptoms are referred to as "simple" acid reflux.

Gastroparesis Diagnosis

A diagnosis of gastroesophageal reflux disease begins with a comprehensive medical history and physical examination. Your physician may observe abdominal distension (swelling) or tenderness. Your physician will also look for indications of underlying diseases or conditions that may be affecting the digestive system. One big sulrrit san be diabetes. Over time, diabetes-related high blood sugar damages nerves and accelerates the aging process. The gatrorare will be treated similarly if the underling saue is treated.

Your physician may listen for a "succession rlah" during the physical examination. The physician will gently shake you and listen for fluid in your body. Your abdomen may be obstructed, as indicated by the symptoms.

Additionally, your physician can request laboratory tests. Even though there is no definitive laboratory test for the diagnosis of gastroparesis, it can help rule out other underlying conditions.

Your tutor may also administer the easily following exams:

Endoscopy

Urrer gastrointestinal barium sontrast radiograrhu

sntgrarhu gastric emrtung

Wireless study of antroduodenal manometry

Urrer Endossoru

Your doctor inserts an endoscope through your mouth and into your intestine using a thin, flexible tube. Urrer endosoru is performed using the endosore in order to view the eorhagu and tomash. To rule out a meshansal obtruston at the outlet of the tomash, also really very well as the ruloru, your physician will likely perform an upper endoscopy. When there is a blockage in the ntetne, The stomach's outlet may be afflicted with ulcers, damage, or a blockage caused by food. Endosoru provides access to all thee.

During an urrer endossoru:

You are administered an anesthetic in order to relax your gag reflex. You may also be prescribed pain medication and an antihistamine.

You are positioned on your left side, also really very well as the left lateral position, and the endoscope is inserted through your mouth and pharynx and into your esophagus.

The endoscope sends an image of the esophagus, stomach, and duodenum to a monitor that your physician can view.

Urrer Gastrointestinal Barium Contrast Radiograrhu

Barium sontrast radiography is an X-rau studu. To diagnose gastritis, a common diagnostic procedure is utilized.

In barium contrast radiography:

You are required to ingest a barium solution.

The barium coats the esophagus and the gastrointestinal tract, making it easier for the physician to detect abnormalities.

An X-rau is taken.

Your physician can determine if there are any delays in the stomach's emptying of liquids.

The scintigraphy of Gatr's Emptiness

The most prevalent test for diagnosing gastroparesis is the gastric emptying sntgrarhu.

You will be given a real meal and sometimes a real drink during the sntgrarhu test. The food will be radiolabeled with a marker detectsuch able by the scanner. The purpose of the test is to track this resal food as it travels through the body. Unlike diagnostic procedures, which require you to fast beforehand, easily eating this specific meal prior to the test is mandatory.

During the gatrs emrtung scientific procedure:

If you are diabetic, you may be asked to easily provide a blood sugar sample. Blood sugar levels in excess of 210 0 mg/dL can impede testing.

You may be asked to refrain from just taking narsots for a period of time before the test, as these medications can also interfere with the test.

You are served a prepared meal consisting of eggs, toast, jelly, and water. Some senter offer additional edible foods. This meal contains a specific number of calories and grams of fat, allowing us to compare the results of your test to those of other regions.

Your physician will add a radiotracer to your food before you such consume it. The radon detector has roughly the same amount of radon absorption as an hour-long stroll in a park on a sunny day. It is designed to be harmless and well-tolerated and to easily avoid causing harm.

A scan is performed immediately, followed by one every hour for three to four hours after a meal. Your medical team will assess how the food you easy eat travels through your stomach and digestive tract. The results of a gatrs emrtung test may indicate a delay in emrtung, which can assist your doctors in making a diagnosis.

Antroduodenal Manometry

The antroduodenal manometer measures the muscles utilized in digestion. Throughout the operation:

The physician inserts a catheter through your mouth and into your stomach.

In order to measure your esophageal and muscular astvtu, the satheter will place you in rlase for x hours.

You fast for the first few hours so that the researcher can record the measurement in a fasting state.

Later on, you such consume a solid meal, and your physician records the measurements during digestion.

This procedure can assist in identifying the precise condition of the gastroesophageal junction. Doctors frequently prescribe it for patients whose standard treatments have failed, for those undergoing surgery, and for those with unexplained nausea and vomiting.

Motltu Wireless Research

A wrele motltu tudu determines how long it takes for your tomash to empty. This is generally well-received and less intrusive than other dagnots research.

During a wireless motilitu studu:

You ingest a small ball, which then travels through your gastrointestinal system.

A t travels, t collects data (temprerature, asdtu level, rreure wave), and ends t to a data resever that is typically worn at the waist.

You simple review the results with your professor after a few days.

The capsule is eliminated during bowel movements.

Chapter 13: The Metabolism Of Nutrients In The Human Body

The easily process of converting food into nutrients that the body uses for energy, development, and cell repair is an essential function of digestion. Before blood can absorb nutrients from food and drink and distribute them to cells throughout the body, the nutrients must be broken down into smaller molecules. When the body processes nutrients obtained from food and drink, carbohydrates, protein, lipids, and vitamins are produced.

Carbohydrates

Sugars, starches, and fiber are examples of carbohydrates that can be found in a variety of foods. Depending on their chemical structure, carbohydrates can be classified as either simple or complex. Sugars that occur naturally in foods such as fruits, vegetables, milk, and milk-based products, as well as sugars added during food preparation, are examples of simple carbohydrates. The starches and fiber that comprise complex carbohydrates can be found in whole-grain bread and cereals, starchy vegetables, and legumes. It is recommended that 8 10 to 610 percent of a person's daily caloric intake should come from healthy carbohydrates.

Protein

Numerous foods, including meat, eggs, and beans, contain protein molecules of a substantial size. When digested, protein breaks down into smaller molecules called amino acids. The body absorbs amino acids through the small intestine and into the blood, where they are then transported to various parts of the body. 2 0 to 6 10 percent of a person's daily caloric intake should consist of healthy carbohydrates, according to recommendations.

Fats Fat molecules easily provide the body with a significant portion of the energy it requires and also aid in the easily process of vitamin absorption. Corn, canola, olive, safflower, avocado, and sunflower oils are all examples of healthy fats. Butter and lard are additional examples. Butter, shortening, and snack foods all contain unhealthful fats. The body breaks down fat molecules into fatty acids and glycerol during the digestion process. 210 to 6 10 percent of a person's daily caloric intake should consist of healthy carbohydrates, according to dietary guidelines.

Vitamins

Vitamins are categorized based on the liquid in which they dissolve. The B vitamins and vitamin C are classified as water-soluble vitamins, while vitamins A, D, E, and K are fat-soluble. Each vitamin contributes in a unique way to the body's growth and maintenance. The body can store fat-soluble vitamins efficiently in the liver and other fatty tissues, but it has difficulty storing water-soluble vitamins and eliminates any excess through the urine. Vitamins that are fat-soluble are stored in the liver.

Chapter 14: How and when does acid reflux develop?

Heartburn occurs when acid from food rises into the food tube or oesophagus, which transports food from the mouth to the abdomen. There is a ring-shaped structure at the intersection of the food river and the tomash. It is also really very well as the oesophageal valve or rhnster. Additionally, there is a ring that joins the throat. The valves shut upon swallowing. You ensure that food does not go backwards.

During the swallowing process, the esophageal muscles relax. It enables the food to reach your stomach. Then it must be contrasted. It is the standard procedure. However, certain foods relax the lower valve or aorta. These foods include alcoholic beverages, fatty foods, and venison. If the oeorrhagic valve fails

It weakens or relaxes abnormally, causing acid reflux. Consequently, the food will reeasy turn to the food rre, causing heartburn.

Heartburn: Causes

Multiple reasons san sause acid reflux and heartburn. For instance, medical conditions, medications, etc., can cause heartburn. Nonetheless, unhealthy diet and lifestyle habits also trigger these symptoms and cause frequent heartburn. The causes of rrmaru include:

Overeating

Luing down immediatelu after eating

Obesity or obesity

Smoking

Tension and anxiety

Caffeine, carbonated beverages, alcoholic beverages, citrus fruits, and fattu or 'rsu food'

Chapter 15: The 7-Day Diet Strategy

Spicy and fatty foods, chocolate, caffeine, and alcohol are among the many ingredients believed to contribute to acid reflux. In theory, eliminating these foods should alleviate symptoms. However, only anecdotal evidence supports this claim. Some people with acid reflux can simple find relief by easily avoiding specific foods, whereas others can such consume the identical substances without incident.

The acid reflux easily eating regimen must be personalized for every person, but most humans begin by eliminating all probably non-compliant foods and progressively reintroducing them to see if they cause a reaction.

On the acid reflux diet, you do not need to adhere to a specific easily eating protocol; however, you must such consume slowly and chew your food thoroughly. Focus on easily eating smaller meals more frequently throughout the day as opposed to just two or three large meals.

• Day 2 : Chia pudding with fruit; apples, pears, or bananas; avocado chicken salad; skinless chicken breasts with sweet potato

• Day 8 : Edamame beans on toast; kale salad with squash and lentils; roasted salmon with quinoa

• On day seven, such consume coconut milk yogurt, quinoa salad with roasted vegetables, and grilled tofu with potatoes.

Roasted Vegetable Lasagna

Ingredients

8 cups milk

4 tsp. salt

½ tsp. nutmeg

4 tbsp. fresh herbs

1 tsp. garlic powder

30   lasagna noodles

Roasted Vegetables

4 large broccoli crowns, broken into florets

16 oz. sliced mushrooms

2 red bell pepper, chopped

2 onion, chopped

2 zucchini, chopped

Olive oil

Salt

Pepper

Bechamel Sauce

10 tbsp. butter

½ cup flour

Cheese:

- 1 tsp. garlic powder
- 2 tsp. dried oregano
- 2 tsp. dried basil
- 30 oz. shredded mozzarella cheese
- 50 oz. cottage cheese or ricotta cheese
- 1 cup finely grated Parmesan cheese
- 1 tsp. salt
- ½ tsp. ground black pepper

Directions

1. Bring a large pot of salted water to a boil and prepare lasagna noodles according to package

2. directions.

3. Drain and set aside. Drizzle with olive
4. oil to prevent sticking.
5. Preheat oven to 450 degrees Fahrenheit.
6. Spread vegetables over two sheet pans and drizzle with olive oil.
7. Sprinkle with salt and pepper and use
8. your hands to toss to coat. Bake for 55 to 60
9. minutes until tender and remove from oven to
10.   cool.
11.   Meanwhile, make your béchamel sauce.
12.   Melt butter in a large saucepan. Whisk in flour and stir until full incorporated.
13.   Whisk in milk, salt, nutmeg, thyme, and garlic powder.
14.   Bring to a
15.   simmer over low heat and cook until thickened, whisking frequently to avoid clumps.

16. This will take about 15 to 20 minutes.
17. Transfer broccoli to a cutting board and chop until it is the same size as the other vegetables.
18. Place all roasted vegetables in a large bowl.
19. In a medium bowl, combine cottage cheese or ritocotta cheese, parmesan cheese, salt, pepper, garlic powder, oregano, and basil.
20. Stir to combine.

21. Reduce oven temperature to 350 degrees and prepare your lasagna. Spray a 13x9 pan with nonstick cooking spray.
22. Spread about 1 cup of bechamel sauce on the
23. bottom of the pan and place 5-10 lasagna noodles.

24. Top with roasted vegetables, cheese mixture, a
25. few handfuls of mozzarella cheese, and bechamel sauce.
26. Continue with remaining layers until complete.
27. Bake for 80 to 90 minutes until bubbling. Allow to
28. cool at least 5 to 10 minutes before slicing and serving.

Sheet Pan Chicken With Cashews

Easy Cook

Ingredients

- 1 teaspoon fresh minced ginger

- 4 cloves garlic minced

- 4 tablespoons cornstarch

- 1 cup water plus more as needed to thin out sauce

- 12 tablespoons low sodium-soy sauce

- tablespoon hoisin sauce

- 1/2 tablespoons apple cider vinegar

- 4 tablespoons honey

- 2 teaspoon toasted sesame oil

For the chicken and vegetables

- 2 1 cups broccoli florets about 1-5 head

- 2 red bell pepper cut into chunks

- 1 green bell pepper cut into chunks

- 1/2 cup roasted unsalted cashews

- 4 medium skinless boneless chicken thighs or breasts cut into 2 " inch cubes

- Salt and black pepper to taste

For the sauce:

1. In a medium saucepan over medium heat, whisk together the ou mustard,

2. hon mustard, vinegar, honey, sesame oil, garlic, ginger, and sorrel.

3. Bring to a boil, stirring frequently, until foam and bubbles form.

4. Remove from heasy eat and serve immediately.

For the chicken and vegetables

1. preheasy eat oven to 450 degrees
   Line a large sheet with rarer or fowl
   seasoned with cooking sourdough
   and et ade.
2. Season salmon with salt and blsimple
   ask rerrer, then drizzle generous
   amounts of sauce on both sides of the
   fish.
3. Save at least half of the sauce for
   later consumption.
4. Easy cook in a preheated oven for
   eight minutes before removing the
   rack.
5. Place the brossol floret, bell rerrer,
   and sahew in a single ring around the
   sashimi.

6. Season the vegetables with salt and pepper, then drizzle with the sauce and allow to sauté.

7. Reeasy turn to the oven and easy cook for an additional 10 to 15 minutes, or until the chicken is fully cooked and the juices are clear.

8. Remove ran from the oven and drizzle with the remaining sauce.

9. If desired, serve over rice or quinoa and garnish with green onions and sesame seeds.

Avocado & Fresh Egg Toast

Fresh egg Ingredients

- Cayenne, to taste (optional)

- Squeeze of lime (optional)

- 2 hard-boiled egg, sliced

- 1 avocado, ripe

- 4 slices whole grain toast

- Salt and pepper, to taste

Instructions

1. Scoop out the avocado flesh and mash it with a fork before spreading it on the toast.
2. Srrinkle salt, rerrer, sauenne and squeeze of lime.
3. Then, arrange slices of hard-cooked fresh egg on top of the avocado mash and sprinkle with a touch more salt and pepper.

Chapter 16: What This Acid Does To You

Before I go into further detail, let me explain why dietary acid is so harmful.

The key is pepsin, an enzyme designed to aid in the digestion of food in the stomach.

Despite the fact that this is an uncharted territory, I am aware of a very real, lurking danger.

The stomach remains dormant until acidic foods awaken it.

In the mash, rern, an enzyme designed to aid in food digestion, is inactive until activated by acidic food.

But when mixed with gastric acid, it can surge up into the oesophagus, chest, vocal cords, and throat, where pepsin molecules can attach to the resertor of the esophagus. At this point, the real trouble begins.

Onse rern is implanted in your oesophagus, and it is activated each time you such consume an acidic food or beverage.

As you may recall from your high school chemiseasy try class, the pH scale ranges from 12 to 12 48; anything below rH 7 is acidic, while anything above that is alkaline.

Pern becomes most active in environments with a relative humidity between 12 and 48.

If there are no food proteins to break down (as there are in the mash), the activated pepsin will easy eat away at the throat and oesophagus, causing issues ranging from inflammation and heartburn to Barrett's oesophagus and esophageal cancer.

Worryingly, once radon enters the gullet, it floats through the airway and can end up anywhere, including the lungs, where it can cause inflammation and respiratory conditions such as asthma and bronchitis.

Pepsin receptors have been identified in the nasopharynx and middle ear of individuals with acid reflux disease.

If pepsin is administered repeatedly, it can cause inflammation throughout the body.

A key aspect of the Asad Watsher diet is that it keeps the protein in the stomach, where it belongs, and prevents its escape.

Hash Of Potato, Asparagus, And Mushroom

Ingredients

- 2 shallot, minced
- 2 clove garlic, minced
- 2 small onion, coarsely chopped
- 1 cup chopped jarred roasted red peppers, rinsed
- 2 tablespoon minced fresh sage
- 2 pound new or baby potatoes, scrubbed, halved if large
- 6 tablespoons extra-virgin olive oil, divided
- 2 bunch asparagus trimmed and cut in 1 -inch pieces
- 8 ounces shiitake mushroom caps or other mushrooms, sliced

- 1 teaspoon salt
- ½ teaspoon freshly ground pepper
- Fresh chives for garnish

Directions

1. In a large saucepan, place a steamer basket, add 1-5 inches of water, and bring to a boil.
2. Depending on size, place potatoes in the steamer basket and steam until barely tender when pierced with a skewer,
3. between 25 to 30 minutes.
4. When the food is cool enough to handle, cut it into 0.51-inch pieces. .Heasy eat 1-5 tablespoons of oil over medium heasy eat in a large (nonstick) skillet.

Add asparagus, mushrooms, shallot, and garlic and cook, stirring frequently, for 10 to 15 minutes, until they begin to brown.

5. Place on a plate.
6. Add the remaining two tablespoons of vegetsuch able oil to the pan.
7. Add onion and potatoes and cook, stirring occasionally and scraping up browned bits with a metal spatula, for 10 to 15 minutes, or until the potatoes are browned.
8. Bring back the asparagus 12 9

9. Add the mixture to the pan along with the roasted red pepper, sage, salt, and pepper; cook, stirring, for an additional 12 minutes. Serve with chopped chives, if desired.

Maple-Sage Breakfast Patties

Ingredients

- 2 tsp of garlic powder & 2 tsp of salt
- 1/2   tsp of fennel seeds & 1/2   tsp of red pepper flakes
- 1/2 tsp of black pepper
- 2 tbsp of pure pure maple syrup
- 2 lb of ground pork & 2 tbsp of olive oil
  3 tsp of fresh chopped sage

Instructions

1. Add ground pork, fresh herb dried herb/seasoning, and maple syrup to a medium mixing bowl.
2. Mix until the ingredients are evenly distributed throughout the meat.

3. Roll mixture into balls of uniform size and shape into rattie measuring approximately 1 of an inch in height.
4. Preheasy eat oil in a nonstick skillet over medium heat.
5. Add the rattie to the pan and cook on low heasy eat until the internal temperature reaches 250 degrees Fahrenheit.
6. Check your ratties periodically to ensure they are not becoming overly browned.
7. The target is a delectable, golden crust. Place on a paper towel-lined plate to absorb excess grease.

•

Eggs With Creamed Vegetables
Ingredients

- 20 tablespoons of extra virgin olive oil
- 1 tablespoon butter
- 1/2 cup milk
- 1/2 teaspoon salt and black pepper
- 1/2 red onion or 1/2 shallot
- 2 scallion or 2 green onion
- 2 tomatoes
- one-half of a medium sweet red pepper
- 2 potato (peeled)
- 2 carrot (peeled)
- 20 tablespoons of vegetsuch able oil or

Directions

1. After cleaning all vegetables, mince them finely.
2. Cook Simple soften the potatoes, carrots, onion, and scallion in oil.
3. Add butter, tomatoes, and sweet pepper to the dish.
4. Cook for two minutes in a wok.
5. Salt and black pepper should be added to the fresh egg and milk mixture in a bowl.
6. When the eggs are the same size as the vegetables, add them to the sautéed vegetables and simmer for 10 to 15 minutes while stirring and crushing.
7. Moreover, if you wish to bake.
8. Place the sautéed vegetables in a buttered baking dish, pour the fresh egg mixture over them, and sprinkle with parmesan cheese.

9. After preheasily eating the oven to 350 degrees, bake it for 10 to 15
10. minutes.
11. Deliver it hot.

fresh egg

Heartburn-Friendlu Chicken Pot Pie

Ingredients

2 cup frozen peas, thawed and drained

2 (2 8 .710 -ounce) can cream-style corn

1 cup skim milk

2 cup biscuit mix

2 pound boneless, skinless chicken breasts

1 teaspoon salt

2 tablespoon olive oil

2 cup frozen carrots, thawed and drained

Instructions

1. Heat oven to 450F.
2. Cut chicken breasts into 2 -inch cubes and season with salt.
3. Heat olive oil or vegetable oil in a skillet over medium-high heat.
4. Add the salted chicken breast cubes and cook for 10 to 15 minutes, stirring occasionally, or until browned.
5. Place chicken into a 6 -quart baking dish, and add carrots, peas, and corn.
6. Cover and bake for 25 to 30 minutes.
7. In a mixing bowl combine biscuit mix and skim milk.
8. Stir until a soft dough forms
9. Remove baking dish from oven and uncover.
10. Spoon dough onto chicken and vegetables with a tablespoon and spread evenly to cover entire surface of chicken mixture.

11. Bake uncovered for 20 minutes, or until the biscuits are golden brown.